T0114022

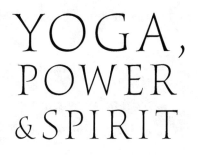

YOGA,
POWER
&SPIRIT

PATANJALI THE SHAMAN

YOGA, POWER & SPIRIT

ALBERTO VILLOLDO

HAY HOUSE, INC.
Carlsbad, California • New York City
London • Sydney • New Delhi

Library of Congress Control Number: 2017942143

Tradepaper ISBN: 978-1-4019-5341-6

1st edition, April 2007
2nd edition, July 2017

Printed in the United States of America

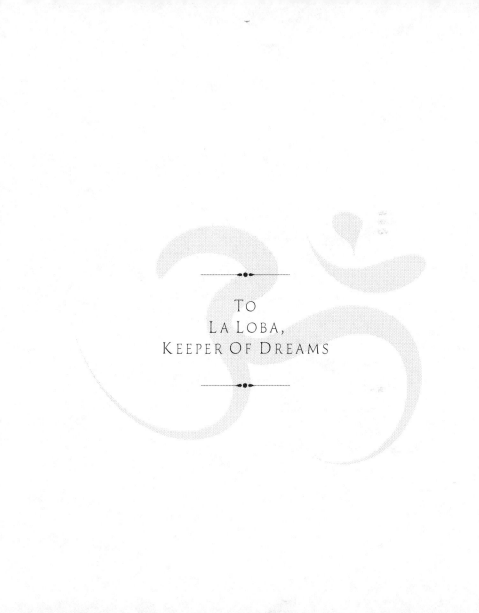

To
La Loba,
Keeper Of Dreams

*Alberto offers a poetic and transformative translation
of the Yoga Sutras that breathes life and radiance into
Patanjali's wisdom in a way that is thankfully different,
but complementary to other scholarly translations.*

— SHIVA REA

*Alberto's poetic and inspired interpretation of these sacred
treasures spoke directly to my heart. I recommend them to
every seeker on the Path.*

— DEVA PREMAL

CONTENTS

INTRODUCTION

PRAISE THE MOTHER GODDESS

The Ganges is born from a glacial spring in Mt. Shivling in the Himalayas. You have to hike for days to reach the source of the holy river, near where the Yoga Sutras were first put to parchment some 2,500 years ago by a sage named Patanjali. As I passed through the village of Gangotri, I observed the sadhus, the "wild" yogis, in stoic meditation and bathing in the frigid waters. Beyond the village I found a secluded spot on the river, and tested the water. It was freezing. I concentrated on my breath, and went in.

Breathe in,

breathe out,

breathe in.

I felt myself hovering above the water, and could sense my body shaking nearby. Patanjali believed a yogi could leave his body at will. I felt free and unfettered, and could see the snowcapped mountains around me, the forest below, and the vast expanse of blue sky that enveloped and held me. Nature and river and sky and I were one.

Then in a flash I was back in my body with a yell that echoed through the canyons. I leaped out of the stream, my skin tingling as if it were being pricked by a million tiny icicles. I sprawled on a large boulder, soaking up its warmth. I reminded myself that yoga is an inner practice, and that braving ice and fire is fine, but the real tests of the yogi are within.

I had come to the source of the Ganges for a blessing from Devi, the Mother Goddess, to compose a juicy, feminine version of Patanjali's Yoga Sutras. I've spent many years practicing yoga as well as studying with the sages of the Americas. In the Yoga Sutras, I found many parallels to the wisdom of the shamans. Both yogis and shamans sought to break free from suffering, from the ravages of old age, and from the loss of awareness at the moment of death. Both sought stillness and enlightenment and the expression of the fullest human potential. The more I learned about the ancient yogis who had lived thousands of years ago in the foothills of the Himalayas, the more I came to realize that these men and women were the great-ancestors of the shamans of the Americas.

There are many scholarly translations of the Yoga Sutras. This is not one. The existing Yoga Sutras feel fossilized and lifeless, the life sucked out of them by a masculine, dogmatic, priestly tradition. At the source of the Ganges I felt inspired to write a version of the Yoga Sutras that celebrated the feminine and more direct path to Spirit.

Patanjali appears to have been a sramanic yogi, a tradition from India that valued personal exploration and spiritual discovery. The sramans (a name that would perhaps evolve into *shaman* in Siberia) challenged convention and did not subscribe to rigid Vedic laws that discriminated on the basis of caste, gender, or scholarly learning. They believed that the True Self could be experienced by direct realization, and that freedom could be attained in a single life-time. The most renowned yogi of the sramanic school was Prince Siddhartha, who as a young man left the comfort and wealth of his palace to become a wandering yogi and later a Buddha. He believed that the priestly tradition and caste system deviated from the eternal truths that were available to everyone.

This shamanic version of the Yoga Sutras brings us to the direct teachings about the mind, about the yogic powers, or siddhis, and the experience of the True Self. It recalls the time when yoga was first practiced along the banks of the Ganges and the Sarasvati rivers.

THE ORIGINS

The Yoga Sutras teach a wisdom that is universal yet must be discovered newly by each of us. Patanjali uses a poetic form known as the sutra, that lends itself easily to memory, and could therefore be transmitted orally. The word *sutra* literally means "thread" and while Patanjali provides us with the wool, we must spin it and weave it into our own tapestry—one that's personal and yet has a pattern recognizable to all who share the yogic experience.

THE SUTRAS

Yoga existed long before Patanjali. In the Bhagavad Gita, written 500 years before the Yoga Sutras were composed, Krishna reveals the eternal yoga to Arjuna. He explains that this yoga is ancient, and that he'd revealed it earlier to the sages of old, who conveyed it to the wise rishi kings. Sutra I:24-26 states:

Spirit taught the greatest teachers directly.
Spirit dwells in timelessness
free from the past
free from the future.

While it's sometimes possible to determine the date when a manuscript was written, it's impossible to establish a date for the origin of the ideas contained in it. In all likelihood, the teachings of yoga come from a far more ancient tradition that was concerned with the question of what survives after death: What is the immortal aspect of man? The Yoga Sutras lead the seeker to answer this and other questions through personal experience.

Little is known about the author, Patanjali. Some scholars claim he lived in the first or second century B.C.E. while others believe he lived as late as the 5th century of the Christian era. It's possible that Patanjali was a mythical character altogether, as is suggested by his name, which means a gift from heaven that falls into the open palms of the yogi (hence the name of *anjali mudra*.)

Patanjali breathed new life into yoga at a time when the teachings had become entrenched in religious dogma and arcane ritual. The Yoga Sutras contain four books. The first one consists of 51 sutras and is the book on yogic ecstasy, or samadhi. It provides the theory and philosophy of yoga. The second is the book on realization, or the practice of yoga, and contains 55 sutras. The third, which has 55 aphorisms, reveals the yogic powers, or siddhis. The fourth book, which has only 34 verses, seems to be a later addition to the original text. It is on absolute freedom, and repeats many of the points made in the earlier books.

THE GREAT GODDESS

The earliest historical reference to the Great Goddess comes from the city of Mohenjo-daro in the northwest of the Indian continent, where her cult was prevalent around 3,000 B.C.E. The earliest yogis were drawn to the rivers where food and water were abundant. These peoples honored the earth for her bounty, and worshiped the Divine Mother along the banks of the Ganges, Yamuna, and Sarasvati rivers. They had an understanding of mathematics and astronomy, and their architecture was astonishingly sophisticated. Indeed, new archeological discoveries are causing us to reconsider whether the land of seven rivers, where this ancient culture arose, might be the true cradle of Western civilization, and not Mesopotamia, as was previously thought.

Devi, the Divine Mother, is the Goddess, the primal force of nature and fertility. She brings the waters from heaven and protects humans. She is the mother, bringer of life and death, holding joy and pain in her right hand, life and death in her left. The universe is contained in her womb. In her fiercest forms, Devi is known as Durgha and Kali; while in her most tender expressions, she is Lakshmi, or Parvati. She resides in all women as the animating force in a woman's soul.

With the invention of the alphabet, oral traditions were annotated into religious texts, and access to the Divine became guarded by a caste of male priests who interpreted the holy books. The Mother Goddess began to be cast aside, as generally happens with the invention of writing. This resulted in a disdainful attitude toward women, as is evident in modern India.

Even the Bhagavad Gita offers a pretty dismal outlook for women:

> *"Those who take refuge in me, Arjuna,*
>
> *even if they are born in evil wombs,*
>
> *as women or laborers or servants,*
>
> *also reach the supreme goal."*
>
> (9:32) (Version by Steven Mitchell)

In the Vedas, Devi is no longer the fierce goddess who battles demons, but is the nurse and lover. She is the consort to Shiva, mother to Ganesh, and wife to Vishnu. Worshipers today bring her sweets and plastic jewelry. The sacred feminine is honored with trinkets! The Goddess lost her seat of honor and became subordinate to the masculine divinity. Later, as she made her way to Europe, she began to be demonized. The English word *devil* is hauntingly similar to "Devi."

Until recently, women in India couldn't own property. Brides are still set on fire by in-laws who consider their dowries insufficient. Even the path of the sadhu is closed to women, and 90 percent of these yogis are men. The few female sadhus are widows who would otherwise be outcasts.

Women around the world are beginning to reclaim their power and divinity, and the Devi that resides deep within them. They are discovering that the path to bliss is not through arcane rituals and rules, or inside dusty tomes filled with men's stories. This version of the Yoga Sutras is a step in this direction.

THE ANCIENT WISDOM

The off-handed dismissal of the Native American spiritual traditions as primitive mysticism is a glaring example of colonial anthropology. We know that history is written by the conqueror, not of the vanquished. The indigenous Americans were in many ways more advanced than the European invaders. In the early 1500s there were more than 125,000 citizens living in Teotihuacán, Mexico, in a spotlessly clean city with running water and sanitation. Meanwhile less than 100,000 people lived in London, largely in squalor.

Colonial bias prevailed during the occupation of India by the British, who claimed that the Vedas were authored by Aryan peoples who brought their sophisticated ways to India. They argued that such a brilliant piece of literature, called by the German philosopher Hegel "the starting point for the whole

Western world," couldn't have been authored by dark-skinned primitives from the Indian subcontinent.

The lore of India describes saints who could fly through the air, yogis who could travel across great distances in an instant and who could disappear and reappear at will. Patanjali speaks of these powers in Sutra III:46

Embracing these powers
mastering the elements
travelling through time and space
the yogi can fashion a new body for himself
one that ages, heals, and dies differently.

The yogi can develop the ability to break free from the confines of the body at any time, not just at the moment of death, and to journey to the heavenly realms to receive divine knowledge. This knowledge is so powerful that it can heal all ills and even grant one a new physical form infused with perfect health.

The magical flight is possible only if the yogi does away with his personal history and cuts the chords that keep him bound to karma. He must become a *jivamukta*, one who is liberated in life. After this, his acts have no consequence, he will accrue no karma, and he will act for the benefit of all beings.

The yogi of the Sutras abhors excessive ritual and ceremoniousness. She disdains confining religious forms and breaks their patriarchal rules. She practices *pranayama*, or deep cyclic breathing; *asana*, the specific postures of yoga; and *ekagata*, or single-mindedness. These practices bring her to the direct experience of her True Self.

Patanjali did away with the hierarchies of priests, temples, and even with the notion of the guru and of God itself. The Yoga Sutras tell us to look within, to practice *pratyahara*, and experience *samadhi*, pure bliss. Patanjali cuts straight to the heart of the practice, to direct experience.

Patanjali describes the powers that arise spontaneously as a result of one's practice, the *siddhis*, and how they can help one to attain supreme freedom. He also cautions us to not be seduced by these seemingly supernatural abilities. Patanjali tells us that these are "perfections" of the human condition. (The word *siddhi* means perfection.) To deny them is to deny your ultimate nature. You can only step beyond these powers once you have attained them. Renouncing them beforehand, as many practitioners of yoga do, forestalls true liberation. The feminine side of yoga says to embrace the siddhis, to flex your spiritual muscles, to step beyond time and form and experience freedom from karma and cyclic existence.

While Patanjali accepts the existence of Isvara, the Lord, he does not attribute any great importance to him. Isvara is not the creator of the world, and he is not involved at all in human endeavors.

He is the Lord of yogis, and can assist those who have chosen the path of yoga. He has no personality, and is neither vengeful nor forgiving. Isvara is pure Spirit, never having entered the stream of time or karma, and cannot be influenced by rituals, mantras, or devotion.

BREAKING FREE FROM MIND

Patanjali states that human suffering arises because we confuse the mind with the spirit and the ego with the True Self. Freedom can be attained when we resolve this mix-up, first by understanding the nature of the mind, then by achieving the immediate experience of our True Self. Patanjali claims that freedom cannot be attained through study or learning only; it requires yogic practice, entering timelessness, and tasting infinity.

At the source of the Ganges River I met many *sadhus* on pilgrimage. They owned very few things and spent their lives walking barefoot through the holy places of India. They carried a water jar only, to remind them that at any time they can dip their cup into the waters of wisdom represented by the Ganges River, and in doing so taste infinity.

The Yogi renounces her attachment to the material world—she does not renounce the world, but her attachment to it—and embraces her impermanence. She understands that she has lived countless times before, has been thief and beggar and victim and pillager—and experienced great suffering in her journey to discover her True Self. Thus the yogi is dedicated to practice the method for attaining freedom from the cycle of birth-death-rebirth within this lifetime.

The Yoga Sutras provide step-by-step instructions for attaining this, for experiencing your True Self, for unfettering your consciousness, and for transcending the suffering that accompanies the human condition.

May you discover the way!

— Alberto Villoldo

www.thefourwinds.com

I

SAMADHI, OR YOGIC ECSTASY

Before time
Before space
the teachings of yoga took form.

— 1 —

The teachings of yoga begin now.

~ 2 & 3 ~

*Yoga is vigilance, awareness,
        and stillness of the mind.*

*Yoga frees you
        from the drama,
        the tragedy, the saga
        your mind creates
        and allows you to
        experience your True Self.*

3, 4, 5

Your True Self knows
reality and does not confuse it
with the twisted tales your mind spins.
Some of these stories bring pleasure;
some bring pain.

All are forms of fiction that distract
you from reality and your True Self.

— 6 —

The mind spins its tales in
*   five different ways.*
Through
*   right knowledge*
*   wrong knowledge*
*   hearsay*
*   dreams*
*   memory.*

---• 7 •---

Right knowledge is gained
by honoring your experiences
and by reflecting upon
the teachings of great books
and wise teachers.

---•••---

--- 8 ---

Wrong knowledge occurs
  when you mistake a rope for a serpent . . .
  or worse,
  when you mistake a serpent for a rope.

— 9 —

Hearsay, like gossip, occurs
when the mind
embraces words that are empty
of truth,
words that distort reality and
hurt others.

— 10 —

In the deepest dream,
*   you speak with your father*
*   who has passed away.*
You travel to distant lands.
You play the flute and sing
*   yet have no musical talent.*

Later, you taste the
*   waters of nothingness,*
*   as all thought,*
*   all emotion,*
*   all sensation*
*   cease.*

— 11 —

Memory is when an experience
continues to live within you,
haunting you
like a hungry ghost.

— 12 —

When you practice yoga and nonattachment,
all the stories your mind creates
through right knowledge,
through wrong knowledge,
through hearsay,
through dreams,
through memory . . .
will dissolve
like the images from a nightmare
that quickly fades as you awaken.

13 & 14

Practice yoga and your
single-mindedness will increase.
Bending like a bamboo reed in the wind,
you will become steadfast
and grow roots that extend deep into the earth.

Devote yourself to yoga.
Watch your practice flourish.

— 15 —

Let go of your attachments
and discover self-mastery.
Let go of your attachments.
Free yourself from desire.

— 16 —

The supreme nonattachment is
when you accept life as it is right now.
Your mind's drama does not distract you
as you dwell in your True Self,
needing nothing,
wanting nothing.

— 17 —

Samadhi brings four gifts
the gift of reasoning, or the ability to analyze . . .
the gift of discernment, or the ability to see what
lies underneath the appearance of things . . .
the gift of bliss . . .
the gift of awareness of your True Self.

— 18 —

Samadhi allows you to break free
from the stories of your mind,
free from the tales of pain and loss that bind you.

Then, only the karma built up in previous lifetimes
can keep you tethered to the
struggle that many call life.

— 19 —

Experience samadhi and you can leave your body at will,
immerse your consciousness in fathomless nature,
even take up residence in the realm of the celestial gods.

Yet karma requires that you be born again.

···➤ 20 & 21 ➤···

To achieve samadhi
you can draw upon faith
or personal experience.
You can remember the nature of your True Self
or contemplate your oneness with all of creation.
All four of these practices lead to samadhi.

The sincere intent to achieve samadhi
will quickly bring you to this state of bliss.

— 22 —

The more earnest your efforts,
and the more attention you
devote to your yoga practice,
the easier it is to attain samadhi.

⇠ 23, 24, 25 ⇢

Surrender completely to Spirit
and attain samadhi.
Spirit is the Supreme Self,
the primordial yogi untouched by karma,
free from desire,
all-knowing.

~ 24, 25, 26 ~

Spirit taught the greatest teachers directly.
Spirit dwells in timelessness,
  free from the past,
  free from the future.

— 27 —

Chant OM,
the sacred syllable,
and manifest Divine
grace.

--- 28 ---

Chant OM.
Let it resonate
  within every cell
  in your heart, in your hands,
  and throughout your body.
Let it transform you
  at your very core.

29

Chant OM,
> *its sweet sound dissolving all obstacles,*
> *clearing the fog of the mind,*
> *revealing your Self.*

⟞ 30 ⟝

Knowledge is hidden from us by clouds . . .
the clouds of
> *sickness,*
> *doubt,*
> *laziness,*
> *lust,*
> *false perception,*
> *and the cloud of despair that arises*
> *when samadhi eludes you.*

— 31 —

The clouds that obscure knowledge
    disturb your breathing.
Inhale
    and notice your breath.
Exhale
    and blow away the grief,
    hopelessness, and fear.
Breathe
    and dispel the clouds.

32

Still your mind
     and all clouds disappear.
Contemplate a single truth
     and clear sky appears.

--- 33 ---

So many ways to still the mind,
    make friends with those who live in joy,
    have compassion for those who suffer,
    delight in those who shine with virtue and integrity,
    turn your thoughts away from those who dwell in darkness.

—→ 34 •····

To still the mind,
breathe in,
breathe out.
Feel the rhythm of your breath,
the song of life,
pulsating as you breathe
in and out,
in
and
out.

—• 35 •—

Listen to the hidden sounds.
Use your other ears.
See the celestial sights.
Use your other eyes.
Perceive what cannot be
    measured by the ordinary senses.

— 36 —

Contemplate your blissful inner light.
Bask in the radiance
of your True Self.

— 37 —

Meditate on the heart of an illumined teacher,
one who is free from attachment.

Be still.

38 & 39

Awaken.
Enter a land free of thought, of worry.
Focus on the dream from last night
    that lingers, moist and sticky on your pillow.
Meditate on one thing
    or another:
    a word, a color, a shape, a leaf.
Meditate on anything . . .
    it doesn't matter what . . .
    and still the mind.

40

In his gradual yet unstoppable way,
    the yogi gains mastery.
He meditates on a leaf
    and knows the complete forest.
She meditates on a flower
    and is awash in the scent of an entire meadow.
The yogi's meditation embraces
    a galaxy of stars,
    the atom,
    the sea,
    the planets.

--→ 41 ←--

Meditating by a lake,
    the yogi becomes the lake.
Meditating by a fire,
    the yogi becomes
    the flame,
    the crackling branch,
    the oak,
    the acorn.
She becomes one with the object of her meditation.
She becomes the red-rock canyon wall
    or soft and green like the moss.
She smells the rose and there is only the fragrance.
No thought of roses
She achieves samadhi.

⇀ 42 & 43 ↽

Two kinds of samadhi are practiced on objects.

Practice samadhi
One with the object
   of contemplation.
One with the sun.
Become aware of the sun,
   our local star.

Practice samadhi.
One with the object
   of contemplation.
One with the sun.
Dissolve in the sun,
   only the sun.

bliss . . .

– 44 & 45 –

Underneath the moist, dark soil,
  the yogi discovers the source of creation,
  the Great Mother . . .
She who gave birth to the sun.

— 46 —

Be careful!
Practice nonattachment
*   lest samadhi cast you back into your story.*
Its seeds still bear the bitter fruit of karma.
Playing the role you have scripted,
*   playing the scene over,*
*   the dialogue is the same,*
*   the ending is the same.*

— 47 & 48 —

Free of attachment,
your True Self
will shine in the purity of samadhi.
Consciousness slices open the
underbelly of the night sky.
Wisdom and truth spill out,
overflowing
in a downpour of stars.

— 49 —

The truth of wise teachers
and great books are gifts.
The truth you discover
through reason is a treasure,
but the most rare and precious jewel
is the truth of experience.

Experience samadhi.
Experience your True Self and become truth itself.

— 50 —

*Samadhi is like a rainstorm that washes away
all the stories from your past.
Everything dissolves and you perceive
only the primal substance of creation.*

— 51 —

When this storm has blown by
and not even the wind and the water remain,
then this is the enduring samadhi.

The ultimate samadhi
frees you of all stories,
all karma.
It bears no seeds.
It will bear no fruit.

II

·•·

REALIZATION,
OR THE
PRACTICE OF
YOGA

·•·

— 1 —

Allow your inner fire to purify you.
Let it blaze
  radiant,
    and watch all shadows disappear.
Accept what is.
Create no darkness, no pain.

Grow your spiritual practice.
Remember your light
    and surrender to Spirit.

This is Kriya yoga.

— 2 —

The practice of yoga
blazes open the way to samadhi.

— 3 —

The five obstacles to samadhi are:
Ignorance
Egoism
Attachment
Anger
Fear of death.
Let go of your anger and your fear of death.
Let go of your attachments and your ego.
Release the thoughts that keep you from seeing
    what fruits your actions will reap.

— 4 —

The obstacles to samadhi
    may lie dormant,
    but they can multiply like a weed
    creeping silently into your garden.
The obstacles to samadhi
    may appear suddenly one morning,
    choking your flowers
    and burrowing deep into the soil.

Ignorance allows them to flourish.

➤ 5 & 6 ➤

The ignorant man
regards the impermanent as eternal,
the impure as pure,
the painful as pleasant,
and the ego as God.

He worships the ego, and
confuses his wounds for
his inner wisdom and
his mind for his True Self.

6, 7, 8

When your mind dwells on pain,
   you are practicing attachment
   and you suffer.
When your mind dwells on pleasure,
   you are practicing attachment
   and you suffer.
When your mind harbors anger and hatred,
   you are practicing attachment.
You become fettered to suffering.

— 9 —

Recalling the many times you have died,
the many times your life ended by the blade or by fire,
your mind shudders with the fear of death.

–•– 10 & 11 –•–

Weeds in the garden
    block you from samadhi.

When weeds are merely sprouting,
    you can uproot them easily.
Enter the stream of timelessness
    and observe as the weeds wither and die.

When your weeds are thick
    and deeply rooted,
    you must meditate.
Only then will they cease to grow.
Only then will they turn brown,
    decay,
        and return to the earth.

— 12 —

Unaware and fearful of death,
*   you mistake the mind for the Self*
*   and rage when you do not get your way.*
The ego bristles.
You forge ahead,
*   intending to shake off your story and*
*   leave it in the dust,*
*   but it tags along behind you*
*   from lifetime to lifetime.*

Learn what you came to learn
*   or your story will greet you like a shadow,*
*   attaching itself to you*
*   every time you step into the sunlight.*

13

As long as the seeds of karma exist,
they will bear fruit birth after birth,
selecting the parents you are born to,
your spouse,
your children,
your life journey, and
how long you will live and how you will die.

— 14 —

Good karma brings joy.
Bad karma brings suffering.

~ 15 ~

Karma is karma nonetheless.

Practice discernment
  and you will see that even good karma is painful,
  for you already fear its loss.
The fruits of good karma bring delight,
  but they also bring fear
  as you imagine the tree no longer bearing sweet fruit.

— 16 —

You can break the chains of karma.
Let them drop to the ground
and walk free into the future.
No suffering.

--- 17 ---

We chain ourselves to suffering
*   when we confuse the Seer for the seen,*
*   when we confuse the stories for the Storyteller.*
Identify with your True Self
*   and the chains of karma will drop away.*

⟶ 18 ⟵

The True Self quietly observes the playground
  where thoughts take form,
  where games are played,
  and the gunas obeyed.
These are the laws of light, activity, and inertia . . .
  of inspiration, action, and obstacles.
The gunas are those things that can be known.
Your mind ponders all their qualities,
  mistaking these for reality,
  for they gave birth to the mind.
But the Self
  remains unmoved by the
  noise in the playground.

— 19 —

Thoughts take form in four levels,
  all finite, impermanent:
  the body and physical objects . . .
  the mind,
  the soul,
  and the invisible realm.

— 20 —

The True Self is infinite.
It knows no boundaries.
Pure essence,
    pure light,
    engulfing the mind, the soul,
    the body, the invisible realm
    with its radiance.

— 21 —

The True Self is the Seer,
        observing all that can be known
        and all that remains unknowable . . .
        the visible and invisible worlds.
These realms exist for the joy
        and by the grace of the Seer.

— 22 —

Upon awakening
the Seer watches her dream dissipate
like a wisp of a cloud.
Empty sky remains.

Those around him insist that the
thunderclouds are overhead,
cold and damp
and trapped in a gray fog,
but the Seer knows they are still asleep.

--- 23 & 24 ---

When the Seer identifies with the world,
others seem mighty and great.
Wealth and power beckon to her.
She owns everything yet she has nothing.

This is caused by ignorance.

⟶ 24, 25, 26 ⟵

The wise woman does not confuse
the road map with the road
or indulge in dogmatic thinking.
She knows she can paint
the ocean by dipping her brush in it,
for she is the sea and the brush
and the artist of her perceptions.

Heal your ignorance,
discover your wisdom,
awaken the Seer.

You gain knowledge in seven stages:
You realize that Spirit lives within you.
You recognize that suffering is optional.
You apprehend samadhi.
You learn to act with impeccable intent.
You grasp how the mind and the world exist,
    but only because you dream them into being.
You leave the playground of the gunas.
You apprehend your omniscience,
    your omnipresence.

· 28 ·

Through the practice of yoga
*   you can awaken the Seer.*
Let go of foolishness and confusion.
Look with the inner eyes.
Perceive all that you have missed.

― 29 ―

Yoga is divided into eight limbs:
Yama: The Great Vows
Niyama: The Principles
Asana: The Postures
Pranayama: The Breathing Practice
Pratyahara: Turning Within
Dharana: Concentration
Dhyana: Meditation
Samadhi: Infinity

The Great Vows are:
Nonviolence . . .
>   *bring no harm to yourself or others.*
Truthfulness . . .
>   *be true to your word, and let your word be true.*
Integrity . . .
>   *do not steal; walk your talk.*
Moderation . . .
>   *use wisely the life force within you.*
Generosity . . .
>   *give more than you take,*
>   *for nothing in the world really belongs to you.*

No matter your name or your circumstances,
>   *no matter your age or the labels you affix to yourself,*
>   *the great vows are universal.*

32

The Principles are:
Practice purity . . .
    be unsullied by anger or vengeful thoughts.
Practice contentment . . .
    be at peace with what is and what is not.
Practice austerity . . .
    purify, reject greed, lack, and envy
    and the endless desire for more.
Study . . .
    and cultivate wisdom.
Open your heart to all that can be known.
Surrender . . .
    become one with Spirit,
    aware of your sacred nature.
Know that you are woven into the
    intricate matrix of creation.

— 33 —

When you find your mind
wandering away from yoga,
do not fight it.
Think something beautiful instead.

—• 34 •—

The greatest failings are harming others
and not speaking the truth.
These always result in suffering.
They are caused by anger and desire.
Remember this.

— 35 —

Master the practice of nonviolence
 and you will be received by all creatures as a friend.
None will consider you their enemy.

— 36 —

Be true to your word,
    and you will acquire the power of truth.
Whatever you speak becomes so.

--- 37 ---

Do not steal
not even a glance, a thought—
Live in integrity
and you will attain all wealth.

— 38 —

Practice moderation,
*   employ your sexual energy wisely.*
Squander nothing,
*   and you will acquire spiritual power.*

·— 39 —·

Practice generosity
     with your purse, your ear, your mind . . .
     and you will acquire knowledge of your past,
     present, and future lives.

40

Practice purity,
lose your fascination with your body
and the physical form of others.
You will perceive beauty with different eyes.

— 41 —

When purity goes below the skin and
penetrates to the essence of your being,
you will no longer be in the grip of
your passions.
Your heart becomes pure,
your mind innocent,
your concentration effortless,
and your inner vision clear.

--- 42 ---

Practice contentment.
Accept all with grace
  and your happiness will be supreme.

— 43 —

Practice austerity.
Remove impurities from your food,
    your air, and the water you drink.
Your body is purified
    and you develop the siddhis.
You see the storm brewing while it is still a
    whisper on the wing of a butterfly.
You heal the sorrow in the heart of your ancestors.

Your strength and endurance are beyond measure.

— 44 —

The gods,
   the great teachers of the past
   and the luminous masters,
   all become visible to the man who knows
   his own nature and cultivates wisdom.

— 45 —

Spirit is your source
and the cause of all your actions.

Understand this and you attain samadhi.

— 46 —

Steady in your intention,
you'll be steady in your posture.
Asana can come naturally.

‹·· 47 ·›

Without effort,
*   asana becomes perfect.*
Stop trying.
Let yourself soar,
*   a bird carried on the wind.*

48

Nothing can disturb your practice . . .
neither heat nor cold,
hard nor soft,
not too much or too little . . .
no more dualities.

All is right
just as it is.

— 49 —

Master asana,
be aware of your breath,
your lungs as you fill them,
breathing deeply.
Deeply
sustaining your breath,
easily
drink in this life force.

⸰⸺ 50 ⸺⸰

Make your breaths long and deep, like the tides,
a natural pause as the breath flows out,
a natural pause as you draw air in.
No thinking
as the tide rolls in and out . . .
your breath in the rhythm of the sea,
the life force naturally surging within.

⤜ 51 ⤛

For a moment,
  for a minute,
  for a spell of time . . .
  your breath may stand still
  as you achieve samadhi.

— 52 —

Pranayama is like a gentle breeze
that lifts the veils blocking your inner light.

— 53 —

Breathe.
Experience the life force
    and you will become steadfast,
    able to concentrate.
Empty mind.

⚊ 54 ⚊

When the mind no longer darts
  from one object to another,
  one thought to another
  a bird alighting on one branch, then the next,
  then it is free to turn within,
  like a turtle withdrawing into its shell.
This is pratyahara.

---• 55 •---

Attain mastery of the senses
and they will no longer pull you
this way and that.
Sights no longer call to you,
yearning for your attention.
Sounds no longer beckon you.
Tastes do not fascinate you or make you wince.

You experience yourself and the world
as if for the first time.

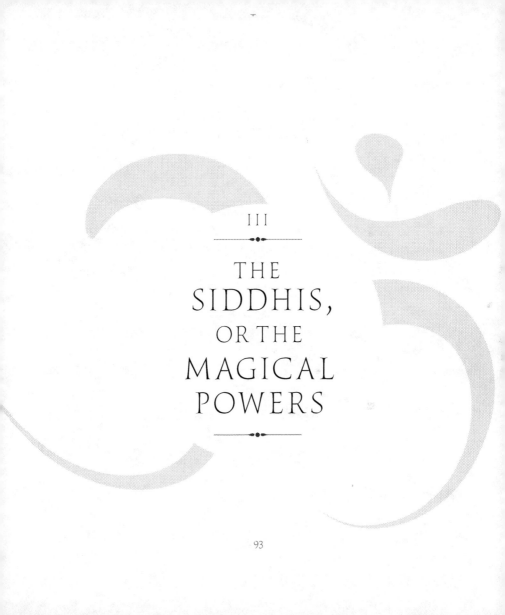

III

THE
SIDDHIS,
OR THE
MAGICAL
POWERS

— 1 —

Concentration.
Awareness rests on an object,
a shape,
a word,
a breath.

Steadfast.

— 2 —

Meditation.
Awareness fixes gently on an object or a breath,
*   unmoved by thoughts that wander by.*
Conscious only of this.

Unwavering.

— 3 —

Samadhi.
Immersed in concentration and meditation,
    all thoughts and distractions far away.
Your focus steady,
    you achieve samadhi.
All that exists is the heart of the experience.
There is no one meditating,
    no one concentrating,
    only awareness.

There is no yogi,
    only the yoga.

--- 4, 5, 6 ---

Clear and lucid, practice
concentration,
meditation,
samadhi.
This is samyana.
Practice this when you awaken,
when you sleep,
when you dream.
Then the light of wisdom grows,
illuminating the way to
even higher states of being.

7 & 8

*Unlike the other limbs of yoga
    concentration, meditation, and samadhi
    are practiced within one's self.
Yet once you taste the ultimate samadhi
    where the seeds of karma cease to exist,
    even these practices will seem external.*

I have ceased to exist.

— 9 —

In samyana, memories rise to the surface,
dissolve naturally,
yet leave tiny ripples in the awareness
that radiate outward toward the shore
until the surface smoothes itself.
Mind and awareness merge
again in stillness.

— 10 —

In stillness
  true power requires no exertion,
  no effort.
Simply practice yoga.
  Then awareness will cease to waver,
  untouched by the swirling winds of
  thought, worry, and desire.

→ 11 & 12 ←

Be still and in samadhi
  and your eyes will open.
You will see the birth of the galaxies
  and the death of the universe.
You may even be swept up in the
  astral river of infinity,
  gulping mouthfuls of timelessness,
  swallowing past and future in the same instant.

13 & 14

Immersed in this river of timelessness,
     you will come to know the secrets of nature,
     understand transformation,
     from larva to cocoon to butterfly . . .
     from acorn to oak . . .
     and recognize the matrix of a tree,
     which resides in the unseen world.

You will solve the riddles of how
     time flows in more than one direction,
     and unravel the mysteries etched in layers of stone,
     ash, and bone deep within the earth.

— 15 & 16 —

Practice samyana on the egg, the serpent,
*   and the sloughed-off skin,*
*   on the changing nature of all things . . .*
*   and you will know the future as well as the past.*

— 17 —

Hear the call of the loon resounding across the lake.
Practice samyana on its haunting cry
*   and you will understand its language.*
Know that it is flirting with its mate
*   or singing in joy.*
Practice samyana on your lover's words
*   and you will not confuse her*
*   speech with what she is telling you*
*   in her heart.*

~ 18 ~

The specters of former lives
   are dim apparitions that float through your mind.
They can be seen clearly when you practice samyana.
Your stories will appear on their faces,
   memories from every one of your past lifetimes.
You will remember everything that you have forgotten.

— 19 & 20 —

Look upon another.
Practice samyana on his grimace or his smile,
    the straightening of shoulders,
    his walk,
    and you will understand what is in the mind of that person,
    but the secrets of his heart will remain hidden.

··· 21 & 22 ···

Practice samyana on the form of your body,
    the curve of your leg,
    the outline of your fingers,
    and you can become invisible,
    no longer seen by others
    beyond the perception of the senses.

Enter a room and you are noticed
    when you choose to be seen,
    unheard,
    unfelt,
    yet in full mastery of the light and
    power emanating from you.

— 23 —

The stories of your past will be retold today
   or in another lifetime
   when your karma manifests.
Practice samyana on the memories of your past lives
   on the memories of your past deaths.
Practice samyana on the signs of your mortality.

You will master how and when this lifetime will end
   and be prepared to meet infinity.

—• 24 •—

Practice samyana on love or compassion,
virtue or creativity,
and these qualities will be yours to use,
yours to bestow
on whomever may need them.

— 25 —

Practice samyana on the strength of elephants
and you will stomp on obstacles as
if they were mere blades of grass.
Acquire strength of the heart and soul.
Practice samyana on the creatures of
the forest and the mountain.
Try on their wings, their vision, their instincts,
until they become yours.

— 26 —

Practice samyana on your inner radiance
*   and you will gain wisdom.*
Secrets will reveal themselves.
You will know about each drop of water
*   and the cloud that holds them.*
Nothing will be too small or too large for you to grasp.
You will know why the rain clouds are not in the sky
*   and how to call them back.*
You will know that there are
*   showers in the valley miles away.*

You will know this because
*   far away and near have ceased to exist for you.*

27, 28, 29

Practice samyana on the sun,
and you will know the seven heavenly realms,
the six hells and the netherworlds.
Practice samyana on the moon,
and you will know every star.
Practice samyana on the North Star
and you will know the heart of the Milky Way,
the far-off galaxies
and the journey of the planets.

30, 31, 32, 33

Practice samyana on the chakra at your navel.
See inside your body or that of someone else.
You will know the workings of each organ
and the health of your body or hers.
Practice samyana on the chakra at your throat . . .
slake your thirst and sate your hunger.
Practice samyana on the hollow below your throat
and as you meditate you will feel yourself relax.

Practice samyana on the light above your head
and you will perceive the luminous ones,
the angels and the masters.

— 34 —

Gradually
  or in the flash of an instant,
  one can achieve the siddhis
  and all the hidden knowledge is revealed.

— 35 —

Practice samyana on the heart chakra
and know pure mind.

— 36 —

The mind and the Self must not be confused,
for the mind is fleeting and temporary
and is meant to serve its master.
When you confuse the Self for the mind,
you suffer.

Practice samyana on the distinction
between the mind and the Self
and you will dwell in your divinity.

Once you know you are a
spiritual being in a body,
a visitor in this world,
you will never again
need a spiritual experience.

—• 37 & 38 •—

Clearly distinguishing between the mind and the Self,
*   you become enlightened in an instant.*
All powers are bestowed upon you,
*   perceiving beyond the senses.*
Stepping outside of time,
*   you experience the past and the future.*
Enjoy the gift of the siddhis.
You have achieved perfection.

If you swell with pride over these powers,
*   you will be held back from the higher levels of samadhi.*
If you fear these powers and renounce them,
*   you will be held back from the higher levels of samadhi.*

⟶ 39 & 40 ⟵

Unfetter your awareness from your body,
    soar free of time and place.
You may settle softly into the body of another,
    seeing, feeling, sensing as they do;
    or simply sail through the sky,
    dipping and gliding.
Master the luminous body.
You can become weightless,
    rising like a leaf on an autumn breeze,
    or walk across a pond,
    leaving your body on the shore.
Free of the weight of the body,
    you can master the moment of your death.

··· ● 41 ● ···

Prana.
Inhale.
Exhale.
Master the art of the breath
and your body will shine
with the radiance of a star.

— 42 —

Practice samyana and listen
  across the vastness of time and space.
You will recall the tales told by the
  fireside long ago,
  as well as the stories not yet told,
  sitting with the ancestors
  and walking with your children's children.

— 43 —

Practice samyana on the immensity
of time and space.
You will be able to revisit the past
and heal the future.

---* 44 *---

Loosened from the grip of the body,
awareness rises.
Practice samyana on this freedom
and all veils that conceal the
light of your True Self are destroyed.

Practice samyana on the flames,
  the embers,
  and the nature of fire.
Practice samyana on the damp soil
  and its power to transform a seed into a tree.
Practice samyana on the wind and the
  laughter and sadness it carries
  in the scent of a wildflower.
Practice samyana on the water of the
  creek as it trickles over stones,
  bringing life to the roots of the grasses.

Then you will have gained
  mastery over all the elements of creation:
  earth, air, fire, water . . .
  space-time.

—• 46 •—

Embracing these powers,
 mastering the elements,
 traveling through time and space,
 the yogi can fashion a new body for himself . . .
 one that ages, heals, and dies differently.

— 47 —

The power of beauty and grace . . .
strength . . .
endurance . . .
flexibility . . .
these perfections of the body can be
achieved through samyana.

━ 48 ━

Practice samyana on your perception,
  on your vision,
  on your hearing,
  on all your senses and their qualities.
You will know the taste of the salt of the ocean
  even while in the desert.
You will know the sound of a crackling fire
  even while swimming in the sea.

You will know that you are
  dreaming the world into being
  and that it is dreaming you.

— 49 —

Know that all you perceive is real,
that it exists because you perceive it.
Then the world mirrors perfectly the
condition of your love and your intent.
You can travel at the speed of the mind,
faster than light.
You can feel the warmth of the jaguar's breath
though you are miles away.
You have mastered your inner nature.
You perceive with hidden senses
and know that you, too, are the jaguar,
the rain forest,
and that you and I have never been apart.

— 50 —

The mind, a grain of sand,
*   the Self, the beach.*
The mind is a single note made by a flute,
*   the Self, the breath,*
*   the wind.*

Practice samyana on the difference,
*   then all wisdom and power flow into you.*

--→ 51 ←--

Employ the spiritual powers
to attain samadhi,
then let them slip to the ground
like the walking stick you discard at the end of the path.
Stride free, leaving the woods behind you,
knowing the stick will be there upon your return,
should you need it.

— 52 —

When on the way, you encounter an angel
 who sits at your table and shines her light upon your face,
 attend to your supper
 and the business she has with you.
Should you become drunk with awe instead
 and find your mind burdened
 with even a thought or two of this special moment,
 you will miss the blessing the angel has come to bestow.

--- 53 ---

Practice samyana on one instant
*   and you will know the measure of the present.*
Your eyes will be open to colors no one else sees.
Possibilities and journeys that no one has imagined.

You will understand that you do not cross the same river twice,
*   not even once.*

— 54 —

Knowing the river and the mountain,
 the shore and the horizon at once,
 and every facet of the Divine, the unmanifest,
 at once
 the yogi simply knows,
 understands effortlessly,
 she is free.

— 55 —

This is absolute freedom.
When the mind is swept clean of all the cobwebs
and becomes pure, like the Self,
a still pool that reflects everything,
mirrors the world back to itself
perfectly.

IV

ABSOLUTE
FREEDOM

— 1 —

The yogi achieves spiritual power in five ways:
By drinking from the spring that sources from
*   his yoga practice in former lifetimes.*
By tasting the special herbs that carry him
*   out of his ordinary consciousness,*
*   for they are infused with power.*
By chanting mantras that travel over
*   valleys and foothills,*
By purifying his body as he practices austerity.
By practicing samadhi.

— 2 —

Open yourself to the wisdom of nature,
vast and expansive,
bringing forth life in myriad ways.
Let its intelligence inform you
and transform you.
Let nature help you evolve into a higher being.

— 3 —

Evolution guides your destiny and mine.
Your nature is to grow and change,
*   to become greater and wiser,*
*   deeper and richer.*
Growth is like a rushing river.
Boulders may slow its path
*   or redirect its flow,*
*   but they cannot stop its currents.*

When the farmer removes stones from the creek,
*   its waters seep into every corner of his fields.*

— 4 —

You are not of one mind.
You are of many minds,
    each created by the Self.
A mind that is forgiving and compassionate.
A mind that is confused and suspicious.
A mind that pretends to know all
    but is only a foolish monkey,
        hopping from rock to tree and back again.

— 5 —

In the hall of mirrors, you are everywhere.
Which is the real you?
Find your original Self,
the one who perceives all the reflections
and is amused by them.
Then you will recognize your path and walk it,
no longer stumbling over your many false selves.

— 6 —

Practice samadhi
and your mind will be free at last,
free to close the storybook.
The tales of terror,
the enchanting yarns spun on
long winter evenings,
the thrilling adventures and promised treasures . . .
you will not be in any of them.

—▸ 7 ◂—

Those who do not practice yoga are caught up in intricate plots.
Some are cast in a heroic drama, others in a tale of suffering.
Their karma may be good, bad, or a little of each.
But the yogi's journey is neither comic nor tragic,
*   good nor bad.*
It simply is.

--- 8 & 9 ---

In every garden, the seeds of karma will sprout.
The gardener may be a man in this lifetime,
*   a woman in the next.*
Today or tomorrow
*   the same plants will grow their bitter fruit*
*   even when the seeds fall from the fur of a creature*
*   who sows them unknowingly as he trots across your meadow.*

Karma will grow and bear fruit
*   when the conditions are right.*

— 10 —

Always
> *you have chosen life,*
> *breathing without thinking,*
> *pulling yourself out from the ocean,*
> *filling your lungs with air,*
> *learning to walk on the earth.*
Before the first cell divided,
> *before you inhabited your form,*
> *you chose life.*

So, too, karma has always existed . . .
> *before time*
> *and after time,*
> *entwined with life*
> *with cause and effect,*
> *with mind and desire.*

— 11 —

Look beyond past and future.
Perceive that tomorrow affects today
  and that all events unfold exactly as they should.
Let go of your need to orchestrate your life
  and your karma will dissolve.

--- 12 ---

Caught in the stories of karma,
*   you perceive past and future as real.*
Free yourself from karma
*   and tomorrow dissolves into yesterday.*
Your hapless stories and noble battles
*   will no longer be retold.*

~ 13 & 14 ~

The form and expression of karma will vary,
sometimes obvious, sometimes subtle.
You may think
you have never experienced these sagas before.
Karma is a play with a well-worn script.
Inspiration, action, and obstacles determine its plot.
You confuse it for reality.

— 15 —

One man touches the trunk
*   and pronounces the elephant long like a snake.*
One man touches the tusk
*   and pronounces the elephant sharp*
*   like a sword.*
One man touches the tail
*   and pronounces the elephant wispy*
*   like a broom.*
The mind perceives as if it were a blind man,
*   relying on its limited senses.*
Become one with the elephant.
Dissolve the mind
*   and know the beast's true nature.*

— 16 —

What you perceive exists even
when you close your eyes
or when you do not sense its presence.
The world is real.
Its nature is separate
from your mind and your thoughts.

— 17 —

Perceive it and you can know it.
What is hidden from the eyes
*   and silent to the ears is the unknown.*

18

The True Self is unchanging.
It is the lord and master of the mind
and knows all its yearnings.

— 19 & 20 —

The mind apprehends reality
and hearkens to the call of the senses
but does not shine with its own light.

— 21 —

If your mind perceived all that surrounds it,
you would need a second mind to perceive the first
and another to perceive the second,
like an endless number of reflections,
creating a massive confusion of memories.

— 22 & 23 —

Pure and unchanging,
    the True Self is unmoved by the mind.
When the mind turns away from the
    fleeting distractions of sensation,
    it acquires the form of the True Self.
Then the mind observes all that surrounds it
    and can observe the one who Sees.
Able to perceive the Seer
    and understand all.

— 24, 25, 26 —

The mind is the gardener
sowing the seeds of karma,
duty-bound to plant according
to the will of the True Self,
the master it serves.
The yogi no longer confuses the
gardener for the master.
He is discerning
and he attains liberation.

27 & 28

Should you fail to practice discernment
distracted by the novelties that tease the senses,
the karma from your past will spill over into now.
Practice samadhi.
Remove all obstacles
and ignore the enticing offers
from the playground of the mind.

---- 29, 30, 31 ----

The glory bestowed upon you
    can distract you from your practice.
Remain steadfast and discerning
        even as praise and wealth are laid at your feet
        and you will float above these riches
        on a cloud of virtue.
Suffering will end and karma will cease.
Knowledge will no longer be distorted by
        the smudged lens of perception.
Limitless wisdom will fill you,
        coming not from a book or a teacher
        but directly from your experience.

— 32 —

Practice samadhi
    and the dance of action and reaction,
    inspiration and discouragement,
    suffering and joy,
    will end,
    for they will have served their purpose.

— 33 & 34 —

Time is the uninterrupted sequence of
transformations of the gunas.
You understand this when you
step outside of time, into infinity.

Observe as the dancers intertwine,
weaving the timeline that stretches from past to
future with their serpentine movements.
Watch from the banks of the river of infinity,
which flows in all directions,
no longer following the steps of the dancers.
Shining forth in brilliance,
lord of the dance,
your true nature is revealed
and you are free.

GLOSSARY

asana: A posture, to be held steadily and comfortably; literally, *asana* means "seat," and it refers not only to physical posture, but to meditation.

ekagrata: Single-mindedness; sustained concentration on one thing.

gunas: Qualities of natural phenomena; the aspects of objects in the material world. The three gunas are rajas (active), sattva (in balance), and tamas (inactive).

jivamukta: A liberated soul that is still connected to the body.

kundalini: The power of spiritual awakening, symbolized by a coiled snake located at the base of the spine; the force of spiritual maturation.

maya: The illusion of the material world.

prana: The breath or life force.

pranayama: Control of the breath; rhythmic, deep breathing that gives yogis control over their life force.

pratyahara: A turning within; a level of awareness at which yoga practitioners no longer engage the messages from their senses, having withdrawn from the material world.

rishi: A sage or ascetic who perceives the sacred; a saint.

sadhu: A renunciate yogi or ascetic practitioner of yoga and meditation.

samadhi: The state of ecstatic bliss achieved through the practice of yoga.

samyana: The state in which one is practicing concentration, meditation, and samadhi all at the same time; simultaneously experiencing focused attention, awareness, and energy.

shakti: The creative force of the Divine feminine.

siddhis: "Perfections"; spiritual powers, such as physic abilities and the ability to travel outside of one's body.

ACKNOWLEDGMENTS

The co-creators of this book are the original yogis of the Himalayas, who 50,000 years ago settled in Siberia and then traversed the Bering Strait into North America. These individuals were my teachers' teachers, and I am in their debt for the knowledge that they so graciously shared with me in the 25 years that I trained with the medicine men and women of the Americas.

During my visit to the source of the Ganges, I met many individuals who inspired me and contributed to this work. First and foremost is my friend Shyamdas, poet extraordinaire; and Vishnu Shastri Punditji, Sanskrit scholar and grammarian from Mathura. Without their guidance and deft deciphering of the subtle Sanskrit passages of Patanjali's text, this book would not have been possible.

I would like to thank Reid Tracy at Hay House for the opportunity to publish this work. To my editor Nancy Peske, I owe my gratitude for her wit, poetry, and wisdom. Susan Reiner helped me stay on track with the essence of the feminine teachings. My editor at Hay House, Jill Kramer, has been a steward of the project from the start. My friend Ganga White helped guide me through the maze of thoughts and opinions about the Yoga Sutras.

This is not an academic version of the Yoga Sutras. There are many excellent translations of Patanjali available, and I would recommend to those seeking a more scholarly version that they consult the very fine renditions from Georg Feuerstein and Douglas Brooks. I encourage you to keep a copy of these translations on your bookshelf. I consulted many translations of Patanjali for this project. Decades ago I became enthralled with Swami Pradhavananda and Christopher Isherwood's translation. I also consulted Swami Satchidananda's version, as well as the excellent, if obtuse, translation by Rama Prasada with a commentary by Vyasa from the turn of the last century.

Last, I owe my gratitude to Swami Muktananda, who blessed me with his Shaktipat nearly 30 years ago; and Don Antonio Morales, who shared the Munay-Ki. Their energetic transmissions were the yogic gifts of power and grace that fueled this project.

ABOUT THE AUTHOR

Alberto Villoldo, Ph.D., a psychologist and medical anthropologist, has studied the spiritual practices of the Amazon and the Andes for more than 25 years. While at San Francisco State University, he founded the Biological Self-Regulation Laboratory to study how the mind creates psychosomatic health and disease.

Dr. Villoldo directs The Four Winds Society, where he instructs individuals throughout the world in the practice of energy medicine and soul retrieval. He has training centers in New England; California; the U.K.; the Netherlands; and Park City, Utah.

An avid skier, hiker, and mountaineer, he leads annual expeditions to the Amazon and the Andes to work with the wisdom teachers of the Americas.

Website: www.thefourwinds.com

We hope you enjoyed this Hay House book. If you'd like to receive our online catalog featuring additional information on Hay House books and products, or if you'd like to find out more about the Hay Foundation, please contact:

Hay House, Inc., P.O. Box 5100, Carlsbad, CA 92018-5100
(760) 431-7695 or (800) 654-5126
(760) 431-6948 (fax) or (800) 650-5115 (fax)
www.hayhouse.com® • www.hayfoundation.org

———

Published in Australia by: Hay House Australia Pty. Ltd.,
18/36 Ralph St., Alexandria NSW 2015
Phone: 612-9669-4299 • *Fax:* 612-9669-4144
www.hayhouse.com.au

Published in the United Kingdom by: Hay House UK, Ltd.,
The Sixth Floor, Watson House, 54 Baker Street, London W1U 7BU
Phone: +44 (0)20 3927 7290 • *Fax:* +44 (0)20 3927 7291
www.hayhouse.co.uk

Published in India by: Hay House Publishers India,
Muskaan Complex, Plot No. 3, B-2, Vasant Kunj, New Delhi 110 070
Phone: 91-11-4176-1620 • *Fax:* 91-11-4176-1630
www.hayhouse.co.in

———

Access New Knowledge.
Anytime. Anywhere.

Learn and evolve at your own pace
with the world's leading experts.

www.hayhouseU.com

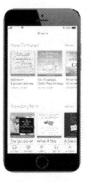

Printed in the United States
by Baker & Taylor Publisher Services